66 WAYS
Caregivers Solve
the Alzheimer PUZZLE

66 WAYS
Caregivers Solve the Alzheimer PUZZLE

ANNIE KATE GASKINS LAWS

Annie Kate Gaskins Laws

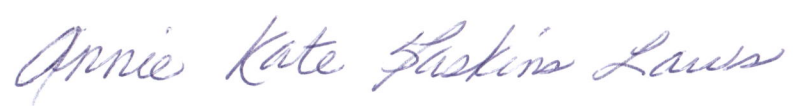

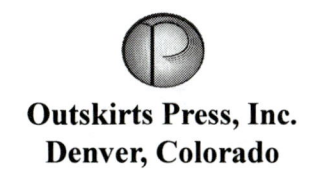

Outskirts Press, Inc.
Denver, Colorado

The opinions expressed in this manuscript are solely the opinions of the author and do not represent the opinions or thoughts of the publisher. The author has represented and warranted full ownership and/or legal right to publish all the materials in this book.

66 Ways Caregivers Solve the Alzheimer PUZZLE
All Rights Reserved.
Copyright © 2011 Annie Kate Gaskins Laws
v1.0

Cover Photo © 2011 JupiterImages Corporation. All rights reserved - used with permission.

This book may not be reproduced, transmitted, or stored in whole or in part by any means, including graphic, electronic, or mechanical without the express written consent of the publisher except in the case of brief quotations embodied in critical articles and reviews.

Outskirts Press, Inc.
http://www.outskirtspress.com

ISBN: 978-1-4327-7445-5

Outskirts Press and the "OP" logo are trademarks belonging to Outskirts Press, Inc.

PRINTED IN THE UNITED STATES OF AMERICA

SOLVING THE ALZHEIMER PUZZLE AND FINDING THE CURE

A guide for caregivers and families caring for patients with Alzheimer's and other diseases with an idea for a new, higher form of coping with problems in life.

Table of Contents

FOREWORD i
PREFACE iii
ACKNOWLEDGMENTS v

1. THE WEDDING 1
   A Wedding Invitation from an Alzheimer Patient 1
   Accepting the Invitation 2
   In Sickness and in Health 3
2. WHAT'S HAPPENING TO MY BRAIN? 5
3. SEARCHING FOR A CURE 9
4. EARLY STAGE ALZHEIMER - TABLE 1 11
5. MIDDLE STAGE ALZHEIMER - TABLE 2 17
6. LATE STAGE ALZHEIMER - TABLE 3 19
7. WHAT WOULD YOU DO? 21
8. COPING WITH UNSATISFACTORY BEHAVIOR 25
9. DON'T FORGET ME - THE CAREGIVER 29
10. DIARY OF AN ALZHEIMER PATIENT 31
11. MY CONFESSION 37
12. DEAR ANNE… 41
13. THE STORM 47
    A Troubled Marriage and a Troubling Disease 47
    If I Had Known Then What I Know Now 48

14. THE CALM AFTER THE STORM	53
15. PICKING UP THE PIECES	57
Reconciling Your Differences	57
Solving the Alzheimer Puzzle	58
16. THIRTY-THREE LESSONS I HAVE LEARNED	63
APPENDIX I DICTIONARY DIRECTORY	69
APPENDIX II A CAREGIVER'S BILL OF RIGHTS	73
APPENDIX III POEMS	75
They Said it Couldn't Be Done by Edgar A. Guest	75
Ode to the Cure by A. Gaskins Laws	76
Attitude	76
Attitude	76
EDUCATION AND RESOURCES	77

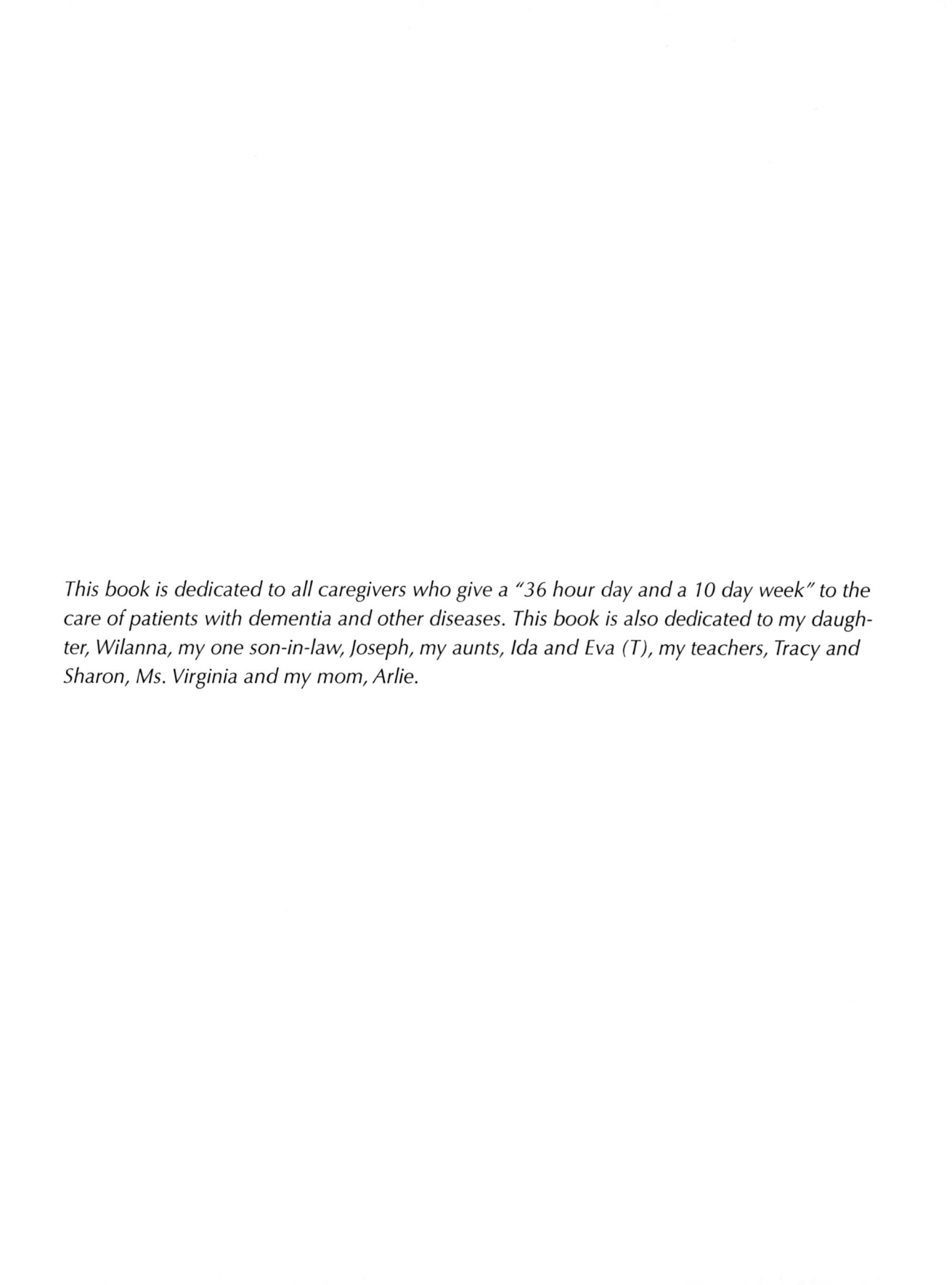

This book is dedicated to all caregivers who give a "36 hour day and a 10 day week" to the care of patients with dementia and other diseases. This book is also dedicated to my daughter, Wilanna, my one son-in-law, Joseph, my aunts, Ida and Eva (T), my teachers, Tracy and Sharon, Ms. Virginia and my mom, Arlie.

READ THIS **FIRST**

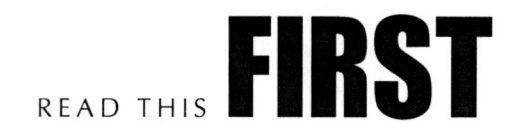

FOREWORD

WHAT IS THIS thing called **Alzheimer**?

I have been living with Alzheimer for four years. Correction-- my mom has been living with Alzheimer for four years, and I am the **caregiver**-- the daughter-- **Anne**. Research indicates that usually a relative or caregiver discovers the dementia before the medical doctor does. True. I was asking the doctor for medications six months before he diagnosed the disease!

Years ago, when visitors would be introduced in churches, community centers, governmental offices, and fundraising events, the speech would conclude with the words- **welcome, welcome, welcome**. Eventually, these words became quite rote and less meaningful. However, my welcome means to receive and greet you with pleasure as you read this book. **I love my recently adopted and adapted attitude.**

Even though dementia is a bitter drink to swallow, I have learned how to dilute and sweeten the medicine. I have learned how to accept the free lemons life has given me and make lemonade and lemon pie with meringue. I have learned to flavor that glass of water with lemons and sugar. I have learned to always view that glass as half full instead of half empty.

This book is written from personal and objective points of view. It is based on data and information from researchers, teachers, counselors, scientists, physicians, nurses and caregivers and the **Alzheimer's Associations**.

To this extent, I have chosen to include facts with a generous mix of caregivers' interpretations and dialogue and the author's personal and professional information.

I want to introduce you-- the reader and the caregiver-- to my new higher format for living with Alzheimer. You may join when you are ready and available.

PREFACE

THIS BOOK SHOULD be a valuable resource for caregivers to use as a reference and as a guide. It will be valuable to all survivors of recent and not-so-recent illnesses and deaths in the family. **I suggest reading the Appendix first - then we will find ourselves on the same page. Searching for the Cure is, by design, the shortest chapter.**

The Two Attitudes are thoughts from poems collected ten years ago. I integrated these poems with The Serenity Prayers.

Many collectors collect dolls, music, stamps, old coins and new money; but I collect inspirational poems and articles. During the year of 2005 I noticed that my collections all had a certain tone - a certain theme. They were all very inspirational. Immediately, I conceived this idea to publish, to distribute, and to share with my world what I have learned.

I have in my collections newspaper columns I wrote eighteen years ago. At this time, I decided to include excerpts from these inspirational articles in my first book about **Alzheimer.** Presently, I am continuing to retain and update the newspaper articles for my second book.

Recently, I misplaced the Autobiography I wrote over forty years ago. However, I distinctly remember the opening and closing paragraphs as well as my tendency to give personal examples.

The selections **Letting Go**, **I've Learned**, and **Autobiography V** are combined articles collected ten years ago. The authors are unknown.

After my husband's death from cancer at the early age of 45, friends and neighbors asked me how I survived. Well, that was sixteen years ago. Now, I can honestly answer, here is the book. After my mom's death in December, 2010, acquaintances and neighbors ask me how I survived? I can honestly answer, here is the book. So, to my readers and to all caregivers - here is the book.

ACKNOWLEDGMENTS

THANK YOU. THANK you. Thank you. I have learned that an author cannot say "thank you" too often. I have learned that I cannot smile too often either. Therefore, in this section, I have the opportunity to smile and say thanks for what you have given me.

First, to Sharon Garrison, R.N., nurse consultant at Alzheimer Community Care. West Palm Beach, Florida Let me count the ways you have made me smile. You were the first person to introduce me to the real world of Alzheimer. So thanks Sharon for introducing me to my first ever Support Group.

Secondly, I want to surprise acclaimed writer, Tracey Spence Banks, who gave me the opportunity to read my poetry in class.

Thirdly, I want to surprise West Palm Beach, Florida Residents, Bishop Granger and Co-Pastor Katrina Granger, who unknowingly provided inspiration for my writing. The recognition you gave me when I presented my original poems catapulted me to writing my first book. Even for me, this book writing was a leap of faith - A VERY BIG LEAP OF FAITH.

Finally, I will say "merci" to my daughter, Wilanna, who is phonetically and physically a combination of her father, Willie, and her mother, Annie.

Once, writing letters was a major means of communication-- when stamps were six cents. Each time I forgot something, I could always write P.S. at the end of the letter and add my important note. So, to West Palm Beach, Florida resident - Ms. Virginia, my mom's former roommate, and my new best friend, you are very important to us. Your courage, your empathy, your health and your smile mean so much to our family!

To scientist, Alois Alzheimer, thanks for paving the road to the cure.

Thanks to my only son-in-law, Joseph Morgan of West Palm Beach, Florida. Oh yes, thanks to the Baker, Bernard and Edwards families of Ocala, Florida and my Ocilla classmates

- Elizabeth Williams, Mary Heights Smith, and Annie Lee White. Thanks for staying in touch.

Hello to my college classmate and French study partner, Barbara Davis Moore. Fort Valley University, Fort Valley, Georgia who unknowingly supported my writing ideas during my college years.

Hello to Rosa Henderson of Fitzgerald, Georgia And to you T and Belle for giving me the opportunity to get reacquainted with Rosa.

Hello to Hosea, Dorothy, Eddie and Jimmy of Ocilla, Georgia Now you know my birthday is really February 13 instead of February 14.

Caregivers!

Thank you!

1

THE WEDDING

A WEDDING INVITATION

YOU ARE CORDIALLY invited to a wedding in February of next year. The time and place are blurred in my mind, but I do know that my son is marrying the girl. Please ignore my errors. I am having difficulty writing. I am inviting you to my world of Alzheimer.

Yes, I want you to come into my world for at least one reading of this book. Then you will know why I am quiet at dawn or why I am agitated at sundown.

You will know why I am moody at times. You will know why I wander and pace. You will know why I suddenly begin fighting or using profanity.

You will know why I am suspicious, and you will know why I say things that are untrue.

Finally, you will know why I hate to bathe, you will know why I asked you to balance my checkbook and you will understand why I don't remember what happened yesterday.

Sometimes, I know I don't make sense.

| What time is it? | Who are you? | Put all flowers in the state. |
| Di de di b de? | What time is it? | Who did you say you were? |

Sometimes, I don't make sense - I know.

What am I doing - inviting you to a wedding or writing you a letter?

Answer me? What did you say? I can't hear you. Talk louder. Don't talk so loud. Stop hollering at me! You are so cruel to me. You are making me cry!!

I know - sometimes I don't make sense.

Welcome to my world!!!
Love,
Alz

ACCEPTING AN INVITATION

I am glad you accepted my invitation to my world. My niece will give you a test to see if you can enter and live in my world while you are visiting. Don't worry, if you answer most questions true, you will pass the test.

TEST

DIRECTIONS:
Answer either true or false.

1. Alzheimer is treatable and curable.
2. Severe memory loss is a symptom of dementia.
3. There is no reason to be ashamed because a family member has dementia.
4. The person with dementia has difficulty remembering things.
5. Little things may upset people with memory problems.
6. The key to coping with dementia is to use common sense.
7. Damage to the brain affects memory, writing, walking and speaking.
8. Some people with dementia have hallucinations or see or hear things that are not real.
9. Hallucinations can be frightening to some family members.
10. Little things may upset people with memory problems.
11. Some people with dementia hide things or accuse others of stealing from them.
12. Confused and brain-injured people can experience joy and happiness.
13. Confused people have the ability to enjoy life and to enjoy other caregivers.
14. Dementia requires continuing medical attention.
15. Patients who are forgetful are usually diagnosed with dementia.

16. Patients with dementia may forget what time it is or where they are.
17. Patients with dementia may remember ancient events more clearly than recent events.
18. Patients with dementia must be corrected every time they say something untrue.
19. We can continue to love a person even when his or her behavior is difficult.

Thanks for entering my world.
Alz

IN SICKNESS AND IN HEALTH
"The wedding was nice. Everything was nice. It was a nice wedding. She looked so nice."

These were the exact words my mom said about the wedding. The hotel wedding ceremony, reception, and dinner was the first elaborate and most expensive event in our family's history. The date of the wedding was May, 2010, and the date of her death was December, 2010.

In six months, my mom's vocabulary was reduced to four sentences with the descriptive word 'nice' repeated four times.

In January she had at least a hundred words to describe the wedding. However, by March her descriptions had dwindled to just a dozen - and then, by May, there were four.

Research rightly states that during the Middle Stage, the Alzheimer patient experiences a limited vocabulary, a limited memory, and a limited appetite.

Mom said little about the dinner because she had no appetite. She even offered her dinner plate to a cousin.

Where was I - the mother of the bride? Oh, I was taking pictures during this initial setting. Of course when the photographer calls, the money disappears by the hundreds.

From January until June, my daughter was the caretaker for my home and I was the caregiver in my mom's home ten days a week.

During the first half of 2010 no one seemed to recognize the disease; they just thought that my mom was becoming very forgetful. She would forget some names, which she would cleverly substitute with made up or funny names such as 'Where is Pooky Pooh?' Everyone would laugh and just believe it was the natural forgetfulness that many seniors experience as they age.

At many weddings, the phrase **'in sickness and in health'** is repeated in a rote manner. I think this phrase in the vows should be highlighted so all brides and grooms can reflect on the promises they are making. I believe this vow is nice for Alzheimer patients and their caregivers to embrace.

My mom's brother officiated at the wedding. He said that one time he read the vows and the groom-to-be instead of saying, **I DO**…whispered, "Would you please repeat that…" Needless to say, he read the vows a second time as the couple concentrated on every word in the vow. Why are you talking about the wedding, you ask? **Well, whether written or implied, the same type of commitment should be honored between a caregiver and a patient.**

2

WHAT'S HAPPENING TO MY BRAIN?

A Word Puzzle Search

The Broca area allows thoughts to be translated into words.
The inner brain is in charge of hearing, memory, smell, and language.
The motor area is in charge of behavior, emotions and reasoning.

1
MOTOR AREA

PARIETAL LOBE
3
SENSORY AREA

FRONTAL LOBE

2
BROCA AREA   **TEMPORAL LOBE**   **OCCIPITAL LOBE**
Behavior   4   Vision

6
INNER BRAIN

Resources
Brain Basics; http:inds.nih.gov/disorder
Basics-know-Your-Brain-htm

FREQUENTLY ASKED QUESTIONS ABOUT ALZHEIMER

She does not plan or prepare meals anymore. Specialty dishes she once prepared, she doesn't cook anymore. She would rather drink colas and eat crackers instead of eating a balanced meal. She seldom drinks water these days. Sometimes, she doesn't even remember that she has eaten twelve minutes earlier. **What is going on in her brain?**

FREQUENT RESPONSES

Take another close look at the chart. (#1 in the puzzle) The Frontal Lobe is in charge of this part of the brain. Activities such as planning a trip, planning a schedule, and planning a meal are difficult. Therefore, the Alzheimer patient loses interest in these activities because that frontal lobe is tangled and mangled. This frontal lobe of the brain is also in charge of reasoning and emotional control. When the patient drops a spoon or fork or breaks a glass, she might cry because it is this part of the damaged brain that reacts to emotional control.

Due to damage to the brain, this compromised judgment does not allow the patient to make logical nutritional choices. The ability of Alzheimer patients to recognize thirst is so impaired that they often suffer from dehydration. On the other hand, some patients are known to ask for meals six times a day while other patients ask for meals once a day. It seems this compromised judgment appears in both extremes.

AUTHOR'S RESPONSE

The Alzheimer patient knows that something is happening but can't communicate it exactly. As caregivers, we can have a nice sparkling glass of water waiting there. Instead of asking if she wants water, actually present her with a glass of water - one for you and one for her. Sometimes, this strategy works.

So you ask, What can a caregiver do?

Included on several lists for caregivers, the most repeated suggestions are:
"Use a Friendly Open Manner"
"Do Not Argue With the Patient"

During the early and middle stages of the disease, the Alzheimer patients will let you know if you display an unfriendly manner. They feel and hear the tense words and thus they become even more confused and agitated!

The caregiver can accept the patients where they are and validate their reality.

So you ask, what does that mean?

It means that whatever stage of the disease the patient is experiencing, we accept the condition at this time. The next hour, the next day, the next week, the argument will be repeated. This is real to her - so we validate her reality - we understand her belief, her altered reality, her altered logic, her altered reasoning.

Resources
Journal of the American Dietetic Association
National Institute of Health
Attitude

HEADLINE - 1997 - Alzheimer Is Irreversible And Progressive
HEADLINE - 2010 - Years Later, Still No Way To Prevent Alzheimer

WHAT'S HAPPENING TO MY BRAIN?

Sometimes we forget what is happening in the normal brain and in the Alzheimer brain. Scientifically, we are beginning to understand it. However, when it comes to everyday life with an Alzheimer patient, we forget to apply our knowledge to understand the behavior.

Remember **Sanford and Son** and the two policemen? One policeman would keep it real and simple. For this discussion, I will keep it simple.

There are many brain teasers in your local newspapers and **AARP** (American Association Retired People) magazines. I am particularly fascinated by the brain teaser in **The Palm Beach Post.** In this local newspaper, Henry Boltinoff writes the **Hocus-Focus** scripts. The reader is encouraged to find at least six differences between pictures. I admit that sometimes I find only five!

So, can anything— brain teasers, crossword puzzles exercise, herbal tea, vegetables, fruits— prevent the progression of Alzheimer?

The answer is in the headlines above.

While the researchers are researching, the next best thing we can do is try to understand. What is going on in the brain?

AUTHOR'S RESPONSE

Usually, the first indication that there is a problem is-- yes, you guessed it-- the loss of short-term memory. Next comes the loss of smell and taste and this we understand. To them the food is tasteless. We understand that too. Who wants to eat tasteless food? Eventually, most of the six senses are impaired. As the disease progresses, more brain losses occur, including losses that affect behavior and emotional control. This we do not understand!

Coping With Unsatisfactory Behavior - Chapter 9 of this book gives caregivers help and hope when dealing with behavior. This is one of the most frequently asked questions from caregivers. It is also the most troubling issue according to caregivers.

It is 90 degrees inside and she doesn't turn on the air-conditioner. She refuses to read anymore and she gives me all the mail and the bank statements to read. Now, she asks me to balance her checkbook and to write her checks. Yes, we are dealing with the Parietal Lobe of the brain (#3 in the puzzle). Her brain is not interpreting information about temperature correctly. No, she is not just trying to save money on utility bills. No, this is not her way of being cheap...

Many times the patients will say what it is not. It is not the money. But with their limited vocabulary, they cannot express what it is. What is it? It is the brain malfunctioning-- it is the brain cells dying and decaying. **This is the thing called Alzheimer.**

Once we understand what is going on in the brain, we can be more open and less troubled. Now we know it is not personal but scientific. Now we adapt and adopt the Serenity Prayer. Now we know it is something we cannot change. More importantly, we don't need to spend hours blaming the patient, because we know it is something they cannot change.

Yes, thirteen years later, it is shocking that the headlines are virtually the same.

Resources
Palm Beach Post - August 29, 2010
New York Times

3

SEARCHING FOR A CURE

I'M LOOKING HERE and there, and I am searching everywhere. I'm looking,
I'M LOOKING FOR a love that I can call my own.

These are beautiful words to a beautiful song recorded decades ago.
At this writing, I'm looking for a cure. I'm looking here and there and I am searching everywhere. I'm looking, I'm looking for a cure for Alzheimer. First, I looked to the Alzheimer Association, the Memory Disorder Center, and the Department of Elder Affairs and I could not find the cure at any of these locations. In desperation, I arranged interviews - in person and proxy - with researchers and scientists around the country...

and I am so close to finding the cure.

- Over 100 years ago, Alois Alzheimer looked at tissues taken from the brain of a woman who had behavioral symptoms of dementia, he saw microscopic changes known as plaque. Today, scientists are analyzing the structure of this plaque in older people for clues to its formation and role in the disease.
- The brain's nerve cells are responsible for the job of remembering, thinking, expressing emotion, and bodily movements. Researchers have learned that a small area in the brain loses most of its cells in advanced Alzheimer disease. As the disease progresses, these cells begin to die and this causes problems in thinking and remembering.

We need to keep searching...

- We have searched here and there, but we have not searched everywhere

- Nancy Mace M.D., author of *The 36 Hour Day* reports that drugs temporarily improve cognitive function, but the disease continues to progress at the **same** rate. One of these drugs, donepizel, was approved in 1996. Many other compounds are being studied. With enough information, chemists may be able to design a drug tailor-made to cure specific Alzheimer symptoms.

We need to keep searching...

- William Netzer Ph.D., reviewer at www.alz.info.*org* reports that a large national survey from the University of Michigan found that over a 10-year period ending in 2002, memory loss and thinking problems were significantly decreased among seniors aged 70 and older from 12.2 percent to 8.7 percent.

We need to keep searching until we find a cure...

- The newest, most controversial theory making headlines in the 2010 scientific community is that in Alzheimer disease, the brain is destroyed not by sticky plaque - long held to be the culprit-but by free floating clumps of protein. This theory is detailed in the AARP Bulletin (2009)

4

EARLY STAGE ALZHEIMER - TABLE 1

TELEVISION PROGRAM: SANFORD AND SON

I TALKED TO the son in Florida about twenty years ago after he finished delivering a sermon at one of the local churches. Guess who I would like to talk to in person? No - not Red Foxx. No - not Aunt Esther...

I would like to have a conversation with the two policemen who frequented the show. One policeman would talk in standard police jargon and the second policeman would interpret in simple English.

In my discussion about the STAGES OF ALZHEIMER, I will use this format.

BEHAVIORAL SYMPTOMS OF ALZHEIMER

EARLY STAGE - MEMORY
Short term memory loss
Difficulty remembering names, words or thoughts
Getting lost on familiar trips
Misplacing familiar items such as eyeglasses or keys
Missing appointments

What is he saying?

The patient may forget what you said three minutes earlier.

The patient may cleverly cover up this problem by substituting cute names.
The patient may get lost in the home.
The patient may accuse you of stealing because he can't find items or money.
The patient may need you to keep his duplicate appointment calendar.

EARLY STAGE - LANGUAGE
Decreased communication
Unaffected speech
Reduced vocabulary
Difficulty in finding appropriate words
Making irrelevancies
Decreased verbal communication

BEHAVIORAL SYMPTOMS OF ALZHEIMER

What is he saying?
Some conclusions the patient makes don't make sense or defy logic.
Patient may choose to not communicate for hours at a time.
Patient may choose to communicate primarily in the mornings or only in the evenings.

EARLY STAGE - MOOD AND BEHAVIOR
Mood swings
Withdrawal or depression
Easy distractibility
Need to seek out familiar people and surroundings
Less initiation and spontaneity
Denial of forgetfulness and confusion

What is he saying?

He may be smiling one hour, crying the next hour, and wildly excited the third hour.
He may follow you around the house from room to room or constantly ask, "Where are you?"
He doesn't find little jobs to do anymore. He is contented to sit quietly.

EARLY STAGE - COORDINATION AND MOTOR SKILLS

Good coordination
Slowed reaction time
Possible inability to drive safely

What is she saying?

It may take her an extra two minutes to understand the task you are asking her to do. Take the keys and the car away from her when she no longer can drive safely.

EARLY STAGE - COGNITIVE SKILLS

What is he saying?

He may have difficulty paying bills or balancing a checkbook or making change.
He may have difficulty performing familiar tasks such as playing golf or basketball.
He may be unable to work.

EARLY STAGE - SELF CARE

What is she saying?

She has the ability to complete activities of daily living with little or no assistance. Shee can bathe, care for herself, cook, vacuum, and perform light housekeeping duties.

MIDDLE STAGE

ALZHEIMER CLASS IN SESSION
SIMILE - A figure of speech in which two things that are different in most ways are compared to each other by the use of as or like [She sings like a bird" and "He's as thin as a rail" are similes.]

METAPHORS - The use of a word or phrase in a way that is different from its usual use, to show a likeness to something else. ["The evening of life" is a metaphor that likens life to evening. And "The curtain of night" is a metaphor that likens night to a curtain that hides something.

SARCASM - A sneering mocking or ironic remark meant to hurt or make someone seem foolish ["I've only explained it six times," he said *sarcastically*.]

IRONIC OR IRONY - A way of being very amusing by saying exactly the opposite of what one means [Using *irony*, I called the stupid report "very clever"]
[Calling his mansion "a humble home" was an ironic remark.]
IRONY or IRONIC - An event or a result that is the opposite of what might be expected [That the fire station burned down was an *irony*.] It was ironic that the lifeguard drowned.

CLASS NOTES

INTRODUCTION
   Alzheimer's disease is usually progressive. It is staged according to the symptoms that identify the patient's declining conditions. Professionals often refer to three stages of the *disease - EARLY STAGE, MIDDLE STAGE AND LATE STAGE.* During the Middle Stage the patient has difficulty following a story.

CONCLUSION
   Since simple words are sometimes difficult for the Alzheimer patient to understand, we must refrain from metaphors, similes and sarcasm. Teachers need to encourage metaphors and similes in writing activities. However, we need to eliminate the sarcasm in our daily interactions with our family, our friends, and our patients. Maybe we can save a big dose of sarcasm for our enemies?

S-SAY QUESTION
   Based on the information above, write a one page essay on the topic...
   In your conversations, would you make short simple sentences to your patient or would you make compound and complex sentences. Why? Is this an opportune time to show off your vocabulary? In your essay, discuss why you would choose a thirty-minute television program to watch with your Alzheimer's patient instead of that movie you wanted to see, Give at least one example and make that conclusion memorable.
   By the way, how did you score on the first test? It was easy, right? It was designed to be primarily informational. Only questions one and nineteen are false.

PATIENT - ARLIE
OBSERVER - ANNE
DATE - JANUARY-DECEMBER 2010

ACCEPTING THE INVITATION
DID YOU ANSWER MOST OF THE QUESTIONS CORRECTLY?
ANSWERS - TRUE AND FALSE TEST

Numbers 1 and 19 are false.

1. Alzheimer disease is treatable, but scientists have not discovered a cure.
19. Arguing only makes the patient more upset. Since they have memory loss, you never win an argument.

5

MIDDLE STAGE ALZHEIMER - TABLE 2

THE TABLE BELOW characterizes symptoms in the Middle Stage. Observer noticed all symptoms except #1 and #23

1. Patient remembered the new grandson-in law.
23. Patient continued her daily bathing routine.

1. Unawareness of all recent events XX
2. Ability to recall distant past intact. ....
3. Continued use of repeated words and phrases ....
4. Slowed speech with pauses and interruptions ....
5. Frequent mood swings ....
6. Increased self absorption ....
7. Little display of warmth ....
8. Need to pace ....
9. Need to wander...
10. Increased agitation, hallucinations, suspicion and delusions.................................
11. Loss of coordination and balance ....
12. Difficulty walking ....
13. Difficulty writing ....
14. Difficulty concentrating ....
15. Difficulty making decisions ....
16. Inability to perform simple arithmetic ....
17. Inability to follow a story ....
18. Need for repeated instructions to perform a task ....

19. Lost sense of time or place - What time is it? And Where am I?.................................
20. Need for assistance in dressing and deciding what to wear..
21. Poor judgment - Stepping on a ladder to replace a light bulb....................................
22. Can't remember bathroom location ....
23. Fear of bathing.. XX
24. Urinary and Fecal incontinence...
25. Sleep disturbances - Patient experienced dreams and nightmares ....

6

LATE STAGE ALZHEIMER - TABLE 3

PATIENT - ARLIE
OBSERVER - ANNE
DATE - DECEMBER 2010

Alzheimer - A scientific definition - **Webster's New World Student's Dictionary**
Alzheimer - A disease in which the cells of the brain are destroyed over a period of time until a person loses the ability to remember and to think properly.

    The table below indicates characteristic symptoms in the **Late Stage** and my data based upon day and night observations during December. Patient exhibited ten symptoms out of thirteen, which again proves that the research is accurate.
    Alzheimer disease is a brain disorder. Patients with the disease gradually lose their capacity for memory, reasoning communication, and judgment.
    Arlie was one month into the late stage when death occurred. The cause of death was not Alzheimer but complications due to **Congestive Heart Failure**.

1. Inability to learn new concepts or to formulate memories..
2. Total memory loss of recent and distant events XX
3. Patient remembered the grandson-in-law she met in January 2010. ....
4. Significantly reduced vocabulary ....
5. Increased use of invented terms ....
6. Inability to read ....
7. Need for repeated instructions ....

8. Severely limited vocabulary (use of one or two words) ....
9. Inability to speak ....
10. Repetition of words or sentences without understanding their meanings ....
11. Total loss of comprehension ....
12. Frequent agitation..
13. Obliviousness to others/environment XX
14. Inability to recognize caregiver... XX

LATE STAGE ALZHEIMER

Patients in this late stage exhibit:
- Little or no memory
- Great difficulty communicating
- No recognition of family or friends
- Need for assistance in all activities
- Loss of bladder and bowel control

To summarize more succinctly, patients in this stage of the disease require consistent medical care. They may not be able to talk, walk, or sit up without help. They may have trouble swallowing and they may refuse to eat.

END-OF-LIFE CARE

Even though the patients cannot talk to you -YOU CAN TALK TO THEM. Remember the sense of hearing is usually the last one to leave the body. You can use this time to share memories.

Hospice and VITAS staff are trained to help you during this time. In fact, you may want to contact Hospice staff during the EARLY STAGE for help on how to care for you and how to care for the dying person. The National Institute on Aging distributes a free booklet, *End of Life: Helping With Comfort and Care*

PHONE - 1-800-222-222.

7

WHAT WOULD YOU DO?

THIS IS A rhetorical question.
Can this marriage be saved?

Magazines and newspapers often include an advice section in their publications We remember the Dear Anne, the Dear Abby, and the Dear Heloise. I remember the title - Can This Marriage be Saved? First, one spouse would tell the story; then the other spouse would tell the story from a different perspective. Finally, this rhetorical question would be posed to the readers: What would you do? Then, in comes the specialist or the case manager who decides if this marriage can be saved.

The husband (caregiver) tells his story.
My spouse is paranoid. She is afraid of the cars on the road. She believes I am always driving over the speed limit. She asks me if I see that yellow car coming or if I see the traffic light? She says the light is on green now. It is safe for you to go. Last month, we did all our grocery shopping together but this month, she refuses to go grocery shopping. Now, she gives me a list. We are both 67 and retired. Should I be concerned?

The wife tells her story.
Yes, I say all those things because he does not know how to drive. I don't go grocery shopping with him anymore because he does not know how to drive. I give him a list because he forgets half the things.

What do you think? Can this marriage be saved? What would you do?

The case manager responds.

This problem often occurs during the earlier years of retirement. However, I will not say to be patient and adjust. There are four or five things I want you to do. Then come back to me in two weeks to continue your sessions:

1. Make appointments with your primary physician.
2. Call your Senior Services Dept. and ask for a referral and an assessment.
3. Call AARP and ask about their Driving Enhancement Program. In some states you receive a discount on your car insurance policy. They may be available to come to your home for a little hands-on driving service.
4. Paranoia is a symptom of dementia. It is also a symptom of other diseases. Often medications can correct the problem.
5. Yes, this marriage can be saved.

WHAT WOULD YOU DO

I often visit Carol in her home. She is in the **Early Stage** of Alzheimer. Recently, I noticed that she would substitute a made up name for a name she could not remember.
   What should I do?
   A. Ask Carol to quit making up names.
   B. Convince Carol that she is making untrue statements.
   C. Listen attentively.

Carol wants to drive to the grocery store. Sometimes she gets lost when she goes to the store or forgets to stop at the red traffic light. **What should you do?**
   A. Get in the car with Carol and watch her carefully as she drives.
   B. Tell Carol she shouldn't be driving because she is forgetful.
   C. Drive Carol yourself or make sure she doesn't get the keys to drive.

Carol follows you every time you leave the room. You need to wash and dry her clothes. **What should you say or do?**
   A. Tell Carol to stop following you.
   B. Tell Carol to sit down and that you will be right back.
   C. Involve Carol in the laundry activities or give her one of her favorite projects to do.

WHAT WOULD YOU DO?

Lynn is diagnosed as a **Middle Stage** Alzheimer patient. You noticed lately that he has been reaching up to the **Early Stage** and picking up one of those symptoms. He is also skipping the tendency to wander that is so characteristic of the **Middle Stage.** What would you say?
- A. Call 1-800-911
- B. Talk to his caregiver and primary physician.
- C. Say nothing. All patients do not display all symptoms in all stages.

Lynn wants to watch television with you. **Which shows would you choose?**
- A. An hour long program that you missed last week.
- B. Your favorite movie channel.
- C. The Andy Griffin Show and Wheel of Fortune

For the past four weeks, Lynn has been telling you the same story that happened when he was a child. **What should you do?**
- A. Tell Lynn you have heard that story four times already.
- B. Tell Lynn he should talk about recent events.
- C. Listen to Lynn's story with interest.

Note: Did you answer most of these scenarios correctly? The better answer is "C" in every case.

Reference
Stages of Alzheimer - Alzheimer Association

Remember the two policemen on Sanford and Son. In this book, they finally communicated in the same language. It is like getting two for the price of one. I have created the dialogue from them to communicate to caregivers:

1. TAKE FIVE DEEP BREATHS. INHALE. EXHALE - SLOWLY, SLOWLY TAKE A DEEP BREATH - AND ANOTHER - AND ANOTHER.

2. TAKE A WARM BATH.
   TAKE A HOT BATH.

3. WRITE DOWN FIVE POSITIVE THINGS ABOUT YOUR PATIENT - SMILE. WRITE DOWN AS MANY HELPFUL WORDS ABOUT YOUR PATIENT THAT YOU CAN THINK OF AND SAVE THE LIST.

4. PLAY YOUR FAVORITE CD AND SING OUT LOUD.
   TURN ON SOME MUSIC…MAYBE EVEN SING ALONG.

5. BELIEVE IN THE SERENITY PRAYER.
   Pray for the serenity to accept that which you cannot change.
   Ask for courage to change that which you can change.
   Ask for the wisdom to know the difference between the two.

8

COPING WITH UNSATISFACTORY BEHAVIOR

QUESTION - HOW DO I RESPOND WHEN THE ALZHEIMER PATIENTS ARE AGGRESSIVE, AGITATED, CONFUSED, REPETITIOUS AND SUSPICIOUS?

ALZHEIMER ON-LINE CLASS CONTINUES

DEFINITIONS:

1. AGGRESSION - VERBALLY SHOUTING OR NAME CALLING
   PHYSICALLY HITTING AND PUSHING

2. CONFUSION - UNABLE TO RECOGNIZE PEOPLE, PLACES OR THINGS

3. REPETITION - DOING OR SAYING THE SAME THING OVER AND OVER-SUCH AS REPEATING A WORD - REPEATING QUESTIONS AND REPEATING ACTIVITIES

4. SUSPICION - ACCUSING PEOPLE
   MISINTERPRETING WHAT PEOPLE SAY
   MISINTERPRETING WHAT THEY SEE OR HEAR

COPING WITH UNSATISFACTORY BEHAVIOR
ALZHEIMER ONLINE CLASS CONTINUES

QUESTION
How do we respond when the Alzheimer patients are upset-- hitting, shouting, name calling, pushing, confusing, agitating, repetitious, and suspicious?

AGGRESSION
1. Be positive and reassuring.
2. Try music, exercise or a little back rubbing.
3. Try distracting the patients or try something different.

AGITATION
1. Listen attentively.
2. Involve the patients in activities such as art and music, walking or riding.
3. Try calming phrases and do what you do best to let them know you understand.

CONFUSION
1. Stay as calm as possible.
2. Try to make your corrections seem like suggestions.
3. Try to avoid all attempts to reason or give short sermons.

REPETITION
1. Stay as calm as possible.
2. When patients repeat questions over and over, give them simple answers even when you have to repeat answers over and over.
3. Accept the behavior - you cannot change it - Remember the Serenity Prayer.

SUSPICION
1. Listen attentively and try to understand their altered reality.
2. Try not to take offense, argue, reason, or convince the patients.
3. Give them simple answers and duplicate keys, purses and inexpensive items.

Resource
THE ALZHEIMER ASSOCIATION 1-800-272-3900

UNSATISFACTORY BEHAVIOR - AN AUTOBIOGRAPHY IN FIVE CHAPTERS

1
"You are cruel to me."

These words are usually upsetting to me as a caregiver. Recently, I have learned to take it less personally. Now I know this sentence is like a name calling word. Now I know the patients are not angry or suddenly upset with me for no cause. Now, I know they may be in pain, confused or frustrated with their situation.

2
STAY CALM

3

Now I know that Alzheimer patients often accuse their caregivers because they are lost or they have lost things. I know they accuse because they can't understand any other answers since the brain injury affects the reasoning area. It was here yesterday - it is not here today - somebody stole it. You stole it!

4

I have an education and counseling background. This makes it extremely difficult to avoid reasoning and teaching the Alzheimer patients. Now, I understand that the memory and the reasoning skills are the first to be affected.

5
BE PATIENT

Three or four Alzheimer patients have said to me – "Slow down and don't rush me!" I do not travel that road anymore. Finally, I am getting it!

9

DON'T FORGET ME - THE CAREGIVER

DON'T FORGET YOURSELF - THE CAREGIVER SAYS "YES"
1. TRY SOMETHING NEW EACH WEEK, EACH MONTH.
2. TAKE TIME TO DO SOMETHING JUST FOR YOU.
3. SMILE------------LAUGH------------HAVE FUN
4. TAKE THE AFTERNOON OFF.
5. SAY 'YES' AND ENJOY THE GOOD TIMES.

TIPS FOR CAREGIVERS
1. CHOOSE TO TAKE CHARGE OF YOUR LIFE.
2. REFRAIN FROM LETTING THE PATIENT'S DISABILITY TAKE CENTER STAGE 100% OF THE TIME.
3. EDUCATE YOURSELF ABOUT THE DISEASE BECAUSE INFORMATION IS EMPOWERING.
4. SEEK SUPPORT FROM OTHER CAREGIVERS BECAUSE THERE IS GREAT STRENGTH IN KNOWING YOU ARE NOT ALONE.
5. WHEN PEOPLE OFFER TO HELP, ACCEPT THE OFFER AND SUGGEST SPECIFIC JOBS THEY CAN DO.

Resource
National Family Caregivers Association

HOW TO BE UNHAPPY

1. HOLD ON TO RESENTMENTS.
2. ARGUE, YELL OR THROW A TANTRUM
3. THINK NEGATIVE THOUGHTS AND BELIEVE ALL OF THEM.
4. FORGET TO FORGIVE.
5. KICK A PIT BULL.

HOW TO BE HAPPIER

1. THINK OF THAT GLASS AS HALF FULL INSTEAD OF HALF EMPTY.
2. WHEN YOU ARE BUSY CARING FOR OTHERS, CARE FOR YOU TOO.
3. CREATE REGULAR "GET TOGETHER" HAPPY TIMES WITH FRIENDS.
4. ACCEPT THE FACT THAT YOU CAN'T DO EVERYTHING. SAY NO AND ASK OTHERS TO PITCH IN AND HELP.
5. CREATE A NEW ATTITUDE.

WE CANNOT CHANGE THE PAST
WE CANNOT CHANGE THE PATIENT
WE CAN CHANGE OUR ATTITUDE

10

DIARY OF AN ALZHEIMER PATIENT

PATIENT - PAPPY
OBSERVER - ANNE

Childhood Memory - 1959-1961

Fifty years ago, my mom's grandfather resided with his son. My brother and I were living in this family home at that time. Even 53 years ago, three symptoms of 'Oldtimer's' disease were widely known. As a teenager, I remembered these three symptoms:
1. Wandering
2. Forgetfulness
3. Fear of Bathing

My mom's grandfather, Pappy, resided with his son two years before he was admitted to the nursing home. I clearly remember weekly incidents of Pappy wandering or getting lost. Sometimes, his son would open the car door and ask him if he needed a ride? Sometimes, he would accept the ride and at other times he would continue walking home. I remember his son bathing his dad in the bathtub each week. As a teenager, I did not know what caused Pappy to act this way.

Now, I know that the risk factor is higher in a family if a close relative was diagnosed with the disease. Pappy's granddaughter was diagnosed with the same disease almost 50 years later.

I remembered five or six times when Pappy would finish eating, wash his hands and return to the table to eat again. Several times my grandmother would say, "Pappy, you just ate - don't you feel full"? He would say, "No, I don't believe I do." My grandmother would make a comment such as, "You are welcome to sit here with me; have another cup of coffee and keep me company." Sometimes Pappy would accept the invitation and sometimes he would leave the kitchen and wander to his favorite chair.

Would you believe that the twenty or thirty times he wandered during his stay, he would always walk in the right direction to arrive at his destination 44 miles away? So, in a sense, the Alzheimer patient may not be aimlessly wandering - he has a destination.

Even though these incidents occurred over 50 years ago, it seems as if it were just last year...
...and Alzheimer symptoms still remain the same.
The symptoms have been well defined for over 50 years...
What happened to the cure?

☐☐☐

PATIENT - ARLIE
OBSERVER – ANNE

DIARY ENTRY, 2006
EARLY STAGE

My mom constantly told her friends, "I am so forgetful."

My mom would not recognize old friends and neighbors at the shopping mall. She would give them a hug and say, "My memory is not too good now."

DIARY ENTRY, 2007

My mom was officially diagnosed with Alzheimer in 2007 at the age of 81.

My mom and I began attending Alzheimer support group meetings twice a month.

Oh, what a difference a day makes.

DIARY ENTRIES, 2008

Mom refused to cook, shop for groceries, do her laundry or read her mail.

This puzzled me then. Now, I realize that Alzheimer patients often lose interest in daily activities.

They lose interest in reading because they don't understand what they are reading.

Mom would say that she didn't remember if she ate lunch or dinner that day.

I would ask, **How could you not remember whether you ate or not?**

This question was not nice. Now, I know that Alzheimer patients often forget to eat all day or they go to the other extreme and ask for lunch every hour of the day.

DIARY ENTRY, 2009
   None

☐☐☐

PATIENT - ARLIE
OBSERVER - ANNIE

DIARY ENTRIES - 2010
MIDDLE STAGE
JANUARY - MARCH 2010
   Mom needed assistance getting ready for church on Sundays.
   Mom would pace for two hours while she was getting dressed.
   Mom would phone relatives and friends daily.
   We went out to dinner four Saturdays a month.
   We would laugh, talk and joke mornings and nights.
   Mom's appetite was good - very small servings.
   Mom described most of her days as *"**GOOD**"*

APRIL - JUNE 2010
   We cut the pacing to one hour while she was getting dressed for church on Sundays
   We prepared all of her clothing the night before.
   Mom would talk to relatives and friends only if they called her.
   We went out to dinner only two Saturdays a month.
   We would laugh, talk and joke only during the morning hours.
   Mom's appetite was fair - child-sized servings.
   Mom described most of her days as "**FAIR**"

JULY - SEPTEMBER 2010
   Mom needed complete assistance while getting ready for church on Sundays.
   We cut the pacing to a half hour while she was getting dressed.

Mom would talk to relatives and friends only about two to three minutes each day.
We went out to dinner probably once each month.
Mom would laugh, talk and joke for only an hour or two during the day.
Mom's appetite was poor.
Mom described most of her days as "**POOR**"

OCTOBER - NOVEMBER 2010
Mom did not get dressed anymore.
Mom did not talk to relatives and friends.
We did not go out to dinner anymore.
Mom would laugh, talk and joke only a few minutes each day.
Conversation was limited - She did not understand half of my words and I did not understand half of her words.
Mom appetite was very poor - mostly liquids.
Mom described most of her days as "**TOUGH**"

DECEMBER - 10-20 2010
LATE STAGE
Mom was admitted to Hospice Care.

DECEMBER 25, 2010
Mom whispered "I love you too," to her son. And she joked with her granddaughter for about three minutes. Her granddaughter taught her how to communicate with head and hand gestures - she laughed and exaggerated all of the gestures, which made those final days quite interesting.

DECEMBER 29, 2010
Mom moved her lips but no words or sounds came out of her mouth.
I talked to her and probably did a bad job of interpreting what she was saying to me, but she seemed satisfied about our conversations and the final day was again quite interesting.
Mom slept the entire night and took her last breath at 2:15 p.m. the next day.

DECEMBER 30, 2010
The symptoms describing the disease are accurate. I decided to give a detailed descriptive account of my mom's final twelve months with Alzheimer. We compared notes and

guess what? Can we score 99.9 percent accuracy on all aspects of the disease except the cure? Before you answer the question, may I record one more observation?

Nurses would ask me:
Is she dialing her friends on the phone?
Do you dial the phone for her?
Is she talking on the phone?

I finally understood that when she is dialing the phone, that's memory, cognitive, and communication skills they are assessing. So if the Alzheimer patient is still performing these tasks, that's good... Conversely, if someone else is dialing the phone, that's not so good, and if the patient is not talking on the phone at all, that's bad.

Well, researchers, scientists, and nurses are 99.99 percent correct in their assessments and evaluations!

Research has provided caregivers and family with so much information about Alzheimer patients' decline in communication skills, and about their loss of interest in everyday activities. I hope I have communicated this very progressive decline by my detailed entries in the diary. I believe this diary represents the average and the universal decline in everyday living with the Alzheimer patient.

I truly believe that once we understand the symptoms and the progression of the disease, it makes life and death more peaceful and more interesting. We accept the things we can't change - we have that serenity-and we have the courage to change those things we can change - and we don't waste precious time because we know the difference between the two. This is my daily prayer.

11

MY CONFESSION

Note:

All names have been changed to protect the not-so-innocent. The information I mailed was a one-page chart describing the three stages of Alzheimer. I highlighted the fact that in this second stage, the patient usually suffers from delusions and says things that are not true about the caregiver.

Naturally, there could have been a better method of communication. As the Tuesday morning quarterback realizes, I could have sent them information about the disease in a more positive manner and they would have been more receptive. This quarterback also realizes that the family knew less about the disease than they would admit. Many family members today know less than they are willing to admit.

This letter was written in October, 2010, and my mom died in December, 2010. I will not wait for them to apologize. Once I had written down how I felt, I could forgive them whether they did or did not ask for forgiveness. I truly believe that nursing these undesirable feelings of guilt, anger, and hatred harm you, the vessel, much more than it harms anyone else. As one policeman on the show, *SANFORD AND SON* says to the second policeman. It hurts me more than it hurts them. You know, it could cause you to have heart attacks and strokes...

Within two months, everyone involved apologized in words and/or action. I spent one weekend with Betty. Uncle Marvin provided a beautiful resting attire for my mom.

I had considered not publishing the letter to follow, but I firmly believe that it would do more good than harm. So many times caregivers and relatives push down or bury their feelings and emotions to the extent that when they are finally uncovered, it is has a volcanic or hurricane effect on nearby bystanders.

Secondly, many caregivers and relatives seldom or never hear about raw feelings. They begin to wonder if they are the only people that have these feelings, if they are the only people that get upset with their family, if they are the only people who get upset with the Alzheimer patient...

Thirdly, many caregivers and relatives may hear of these feelings of discord, of anger, of discontentment, but these are so "sugar coated" that they don't even see themselves or their emotions...

So they push these feelings down even more...

Until they explode!!!!

- I assure you that writing these letters is cathartic.
- I assure you that most of these letters should not be mailed.
- I assure you that most letters of this type should be continuously revised so that there is no need to mail them.
- I assure you that with e-mail, My Space, and Facebook, never write anything that might someday embarrass you.
- I assure you that these feelings are natural.

◻◻◻

MY CONFESSION OCTOBER 2010

PLEASE READ THE INFORMATION I AM SENDING YOU.

SINCE MY MOM HAS DELUSIONS - She really believes in her mind that certain things are happening for real and that her daughter is mean to her - THAT'S NOT O.K.

BUT THEN SHE IS ENTERING THE SECOND STAGE OF DEMENTIA WHEN SHE ACCUSES, HITS, SCREAMS AND CRIES BECAUSE SHE REALLY BELIEVES THESE THINGS ARE HAPPENING FOR REAL -
WHAT'S YOUR EXCUSE?
IN JANUARY MS. GINA TALKED ABOUT HOW HER SON WAS MISTREATING HER FOR MONTHS - WHILE IN HER GOOD MIND, MOTHER KNEW IT WAS ALL FALSE.
IN MAY, MOTHER RICHARDSON TALKED BADLY ABOUT HER TWO DAUGHTERS

MY CONFESSION

FOR MONTHS. IN HER CONFUSED STATE OF MIND, MOTHER AGREED WITH HER.

Oh yes, my daughter said her grandmother can be very convincing. Well, she's smart and she is CONFUSED. It is OK to listen and console - but to convict without hearing both sides - there really should not be any sides. Taking sides for or against caregivers is almost unforgivable!

IT IS A SHAME THAT ONE IN-LAW SEPARATES AND DIVIDES THE ENTIRE FAMILY. But the greater shame is that you - BETTY AND MARVIN - believe her. And the greatest shame is that all of this was done secretly behind my back!!! THIS IS ALMOST UNFORGIVABLE!!!! BEGINNING ON OCTOBER 16, IF YOU HAVE ANY CONCERNS ABOUT HOW I CARE FOR MY MOM, PLEASE TALK TO ME FIRST!!!!

It's hard to accept that for weeks - no months - in my mom's demented and sick state of mind-- ALZHEIMER'S, she has been calling Betty and Marvin and telling them that Katie is crazy.

FOR BETTY, MARVIN AND UNCLE THOMAS TO BELIEVE EVERYTHING WITHOUT EVER TALKING TO KATIE ABOUT IT IS ALMOST UNFORGIVABLE.

My mom, in her confused state of mind, has said cruel and crazy things about you within the last six months, but I always encourage her to be positive and to give each one of you the benefit of the doubt. But you didn't give me the benefit of the doubt.

Mother encouraged you to choose sides. SHE HAS ALZHEIMER'S DISEASE! WHAT'S YOUR EXCUSE?

LET'S SEE - what has Katie done--- spent two years cooking and cleaning and listening to some of your garbage - never defending herself, never talking behind her mom's back about how cruel and crazy she is - never complaining - even helping her with her dirty diapers. Oh yes and singing GOD SEES THE BEST IN ME WHEN EVERYONE ELSE AROUND ME (aunts and uncles) - only see the worst in me. YOU SHOULD ALL KISS THE GROUND I WALK ON...

--ANNE

12

DEAR ANNE...

ANNE ANSWERS TROUBLING questions about Alzheimer.

All letters are based on real-life conversations with caregivers. All answers are based on real-life experiences, research, and recommended readings from Alzheimer Associations.

☐☐☐

Dear Anne...
I am sure you have made a few mistakes. Would you share with us two or three mistakes you have made as an Alzheimer caregiver?

Mistakes, I have made a few. Four or five come to my mind immediately:

1. During the first year and before the diagnosis, I wrongly assumed that my mom was aging gently. Maybe some precious treatment time was lost? Definitely, some understanding time was lost. Research indicates that many relatives and caregivers make this mistake.
2. Before the doctor diagnosed my mom with Alzheimer, I lost four or five precious weeks before I called the local Alzheimer Association and joined a support group. It is never too early to call for help.
3. All the literature suggests that caregivers refrain from the word 'Remember' the phrase, "Don't you remember?" and the exclamation, "I can't believe you don't remember when..." Initially, I constantly used these words and phrases before I joined the support group. The truth is - They don't remember!
4. Before the diagnosis, I would cut the visit short or leave the premises or go into

another room when my Mom's behavior was unsatisfactory. Sometimes, I would try to be logical and reason with her, but I never argued!

Well, since I believed this was the old age stage, I managed to get one out of six correct. During my career, I spent years in teaching, counseling, and case management. My whole life was based on order, logic, reasoning, positive thinking and self help. Now I know that all these words and concepts are counter-productive to the disease.

I did not educate my mom's closest relatives and friends about the disease during each stage that she reached. I wrongly assumed that they knew more about the disease than they did. Yes, from 2007-2010 I learned volumes!

Many times, I could not apply the tips, the recommendations and the guidelines to my situation unless there were examples. That's why I wrote the book and that's why I employed the two policemen on Sanford and Son - one to deliver the message - one to "keep it real."

Dear Anne...
To follow up on the information you just revealed, why did you have problems applying the tips to your specific situation?

Well, unfortunately, I did not have the two policemen to interpret for me.

Seriously though, one tip states that the first thing to go is the memory. Or Alzheimer patients have memory loss during the Early Stage of the disease. Oh, so that's why they argue—because, to them, the incident never existed.

Oh, my mom forgot names, people, places, and relationships. Yes, she remembered two of her best friends from forty years ago but not the third best friend.

I'm learning.

Silently, I said, "How can you remember two of your best friends and not remember the third best friend, whom you once talked about all the time?" Several times I would ask, "Have you heard from Kathy this week?" My mom would always give an excuse concerning why she wasn't calling Kathy. Now, I realize that mom remembered this best friend but not any details about her. Everything except her name had been wiped from her memory.

Once I realized that I could not fix this memory, I forgot the third best friend too.

I forgot to call her when mom was hospitalized. I forgot to ask about this friend each week. I forgot to place her name on the program as a lifelong friend. I forgot... I forgot...

Maybe, this demonstrates the EMPATHY that I talk about in this book.

Maybe, after three years, I have learned to enter my mom's world of Alzheimer. Here is another incident:

During the last four weeks, my mom remembered only the two nurses, her god-daughter and me.

Her nurses from last week. Recent? YES -

Me-the nurse from last week. Recent? YES -

Her god-daughter?

She was remembering this god-daughter from ancient history (30 years ago). She could even recall her correct telephone number from that period. The god-daughter had three new phone numbers since this old one was disconnected 30 years ago.

Then I read that sometimes the Alzheimer patient will recall isolated distant memories during the Late Stage. It took me days to piece this together. Now, you know.

Did I remember to insert her name on the program as a lifelong god-daughter? YES

Yes, the Alzheimer brain is very complicated. That is the reason I am sharing these stories. This sharing of real incidents may help readers, researchers, and caregivers solve the puzzle and find the cure.

DEAR Anne…

My grandfather was diagnosed with Alzheimer when he was 65. Recently, I heard that my second cousin has been diagnosed with the disease. It seems that this disease runs in our family. I am in my 60s. What should I be doing to prevent it from attacking me?

Thanks for the question.

There are several risk factors for developing Alzheimer, including age and heredity. Since your grandfather and cousin are not first generation relatives, there is no greater hereditary risk to you than usual. However, since you are in your 60s, age is the main risk factor to consider. The average diagnosis is at age 80. When the risk increases to 1 in 5, you may want to contact your local agency on aging for further information. Be aware of the early symptoms like memory loss, forgetfulness and confusion. Enjoy your life and continue scheduling appointments with your physician on a regular basis.

DEAR Anne…

My mother says she wants to go live in the nursing home where one of her friends stays. My mother is over 65 but she did not physically qualify for the nursing home. What would you say or do in this situation?

66 WAYS CAREGIVERS SOLVE THE ALZHEIMER PUZZLE

I have learned a few facts about nursing homes in general. So, my answer is addressed to all my readers:
1. Patients must qualify financially, physically, and mentally.
2. Learn the difference between Medicare and Medicaid.
3. Learn all you can about your mother's health insurance policy.

Ideally this activity should begin before there is an urgent need for nursing home care.

DEAR Anne...

My mother said she wanted to move in with me and my family. She told friends that she was moving in with her granddaughter. Anne, I am her oldest daughter! First, mother tried to take the cordless phone with her each time she left the home. When she realized she couldn't take it, she got mad and said, "What are you doing to me?" Then she said, "I am so turned around over here." Once I awakened and she was falling out of the front door thinking it was the bathroom door. When I would holler and try to get her to turn around, she would ignore me. She seemed to be in another world. When both of us are sitting in the kitchen or the bedroom reading, she talks all the time and I can't read or concentrate on what I am reading. Oh yes, she follows me to the bathroom door when I excuse myself for four or five minutes. HELP!

DEAR CAREGIVER,

You have brought up several issues here. You are correct. She is in another world - her world of Alzheimer. First, I suggest that you call the local Alzheimer Association in your area and ask for information. Seriously consider joining a Support Group. Check your local telephone directory for services and programs or to find the chapter nearest you. You may also call The National Alzheimer Association at 202-393-7737. Be sure to ask them to recommend books for caregivers. You may also check your local library for related information. You will find answers to your questions in your reading and in your support groups. Right now, the need to follow you around is primarily because she wants her loved ones nearby at all times. Many of the library resources suggest ways to handle this behavior.

DEAR Anne...

When my daughter came home from work one day, my father grabbed her at the door and told her that I was mean to her and that I leave her home alone all of the time. Last week we talked about the neighbor next door painting her home and just yesterday he said,

"No, the neighbor painted and built a new house in the same week."

DEAR CAREGIVER,

Alzheimer patients are often confused. Sometimes they suffer from delusions - believing false things are true. The best idea is to listen to them attentively. Let them tell their stories without your correcting them or arguing with them. Most libraries and Alzheimer Associations have extensive information on Hallucinations and Delusions. Also, much information is available on the internet. Most people do not like to be corrected all the time either. Hopefully, in a minute or two or three, he will skip to a more pleasant subject. Or you can engage him in a different subject, or you may even want to play his favorite music after such an encounter with delusions. **Don't fret the small stuff!**

DEAR Anne…

My mother has been diagnosed with Early Stage Alzheimer. My family physician suggests that she can be left alone for two or three hours at home. Last week I was gone for about an hour and when I returned home, mother was standing outside on the front lawn instead of in the living room looking at her favorite shows on television. Should I be concerned about her wandering away from home and getting lost?

DEAR CAREGIVER,

Many times, Alzheimer patients are confused about location and space. Sometimes closed spaces such as a living room scare them. Often, this happens when they are alone for more than 15 minutes. By all means, talk to her physician about this incident. Keep watching her carefully and if she begins to wander, call the Alzheimer Association in your area and ask about ID bracelets and other safety measures for the home. Also, they have volumes of information about other resources, and respite care.

DEAR Anne

My husband is at the End-Stage of Alzheimer. What should I be doing now?

This is a great question.

My answer is very general. I hope it benefits readers, family members and caregivers who read this book. If your husband or family member is not yet under the care of Hospice or **VITAS**, that will be a great place to begin. When you call Hospice, ask for the bereavement chaplain. This excellent organization talks with patients and their families before death. They continue this relationship for several weeks or several months after death. Your local

Alzheimer Association has specific information about this service. You can find Hospice listed in your local telephone directory or you can call your Senior Services or Elder Care office in your county or state.

□□□

Anne SHARES HER TELEPHONE CALLS…

In February, 2010, an acquaintance called me and said that she hated her mother for all the terrible things she has said to her and all the violent physical outbursts she has inflicted on her. Fortunately, the mother is presently living with her son. **Saying, "Don't hate your mother," was not the answer she needed.** I suggested that she join an Alzheimer Support Group in her city.

I immediately called the local Alzheimer Association on her behalf. Having these feelings are natural, to talk about these feelings is therapeutic, but it is not natural to harbor these bitter feelings and feel completely helpless in this situation. This letter is highlighted in the *Picking up the Pieces* **section of this book.**

On March 09, 2010, I put this book on hold to talk to an old friend who said that after two years he could not cope with his wife's death and that he couldn't get rid of the guilt. **Saying, "Don't feel guilty" was not the answer he needed from me.** However, I did encourage him to call Hospice.

Bereavement is a journey. Whether the spouse or caregiver is suffering from death due to cancer, Alzheimer, or other diseases, the grieving is similar.

13

THE STORM

A Troubled Marriage
A Troubled Disease

ALZHEIMER ONLINE CLASS CONCLUDES

RECIPE TO MAKE A TROUBLED MARRIAGE

Money	Communication	Hate
Unemployment	High sodium broth	Fear
Cooperation	Understanding	Listening
Patience	Ice Cream	Food

DIRECTIONS

Mix all ingredients disproportionately and without measuring.

Add a generous amount of arguing, revenge, blaming, forgetfulness, anxiety and agitation, aggressiveness and assertiveness, wandering and wondering and you have a perfect recipe for a troubled marriage and a troubling disease.

Alzheimer is a brain disease that eventually robs the patient of simple math skills, language skills, memory aids and even a simple smile. Today, the disease is incurable.

WHAT IS OUR INNER CURE?

While we are waiting for the cure, we can measure the above ingredients proportionately and receive some solace from chapter 14: The Calm After the Storm. We can Pick up the Pieces from chapter 15. We can turn to the Appendix and believe that it can be done - that it can be cured. While we are waiting we can change our attitude as we learn more about the disease through our references, our resources and our Alzheimer support groups. Remember in the 50's and 60's, they thought polio could not be cured!

FINALLY, LET'S SPRINKLE OUR SUCCESS WITH A MEASURED TREAT OF ICE CREAM THAT'S IN THE BAG.

IF I HAD KNOWN THEN WHAT I KNOW NOW

"If you knew then what you know now would you have done things differently?"

Nine out of ten of the respondents on television shows or in local conferences answered with a resounding "Yes."

When a relative or friend comes home after an eye injury, or a hand injury or a leg injury, we can visibly see the change. However, we can't visibly see the bandages around the brain, when that relative or friend comes home with a brain injury. We tend to forget the symptoms of the illness and thus we sometimes behave badly. That's acceptable, as long as we learn from our errors and accept that we are indeed human.

Several times during this **Early Stage** I was aware of my mom's symptoms but since I did not see the malfunctioning brain, I was remiss.

I wish I knew then what I know now. Now, I have empathy; then I had sympathy. Now I am able to almost totally immerse my brain in the world of Alzheimer and begin to understand that the patient's brain and communicative skills are similar to that of a two- or four-year-old. Remember, the terrible twos?...and we had a difficult time handling the behavior then!

Remember the child at three and four, when he would say "I hate you," or "You're always mean to me." Research documents results which indicate Alzheimer patients often repeat the identical sentences word for word. We know now that both the young child and the adult use these conclusions to express their dissatisfaction with their immediate situation.

The child's vocabulary has not developed to the extent that he could express himself adequately. Likewise, the Alzheimer patient brain which was once mature has declined to a childish level.

One day my mom said, "You are so mean to me." Even though I know a lot about the disease, this remark really upset me...Then, in January, 2011, as I was reading **The 36 Hour Day: Problems of Behavior (chapter 7) I read the exact sentence written by authors, Mace and Rabins!** In addition to being relieved and validated, I sarcastically said;

"Now, you tell me. Where were you when I needed you most?"

IF I HAD KNOWN THEN WHAT I KNOW NOW...

Yes, I would say and do things differently.

So the patient is walking around with a tangled and decayed brain trying to make sense of everything and everyone in his world and not doing such a good job of it. No wonder he is frustrated.

Now, I'm getting it!

In 2004-2006, I resided in a 55+ community and a neighbor would have a gentle, spiritual conversation with me one minute, but when another neighbor walked by, she'd make the statement:

"I feel like pulling off my shoes and hitting her."

This same conversation was replayed seven or eight times a year.

In the same community, a retired science teacher would perform magnificently when instructing students. However, when a neighbor asked her what were the theories involved, she would become very confused or explain the theory poorly. I would like to conclude this segment by reiterating: If I had known then what I know now....

A few months ago the obituary of one of my mom's acquaintances was in the newspaper. This obituary triggered negative reminders for her. When the new maintenance man mentioned how he grew up with her children, and what a nice person she was to be around., my mom agreed but continued by mentioning all sorts of negative things about her. I know now that in the **Early Stage**, Alzheimer patients often have inappropriate false opinions, make irrelevant statements and use poor judgment.

Of course, then I was busy trying to think of some comments or some diversion, some statement, some explanation, to convey that my mom's conversation and remarks were very inappropriate.

Well, I did nothing then except to "grin and bear it." That was then...

Now, I can give them the card which explains the behavior very succinctly. Your local Alzheimer Association usually distributes these business informational cards free of charge. I learned from the Alzheimer Association that the greatest need of all patients is to feel appreciated. Here is my personal story.

I learned that in the **Early Stage**, the patient has the tendency to keep the caregiver near at all times. So, I thought I was ready for this behavior pattern. I would announce that I was going to the bedroom to make a phone call or I was going to the kitchen to put away the groceries. My mom would not call my name, but she would get up and look for me or knock on the door to see if I was still there seven minutes later. No, I was not ready for this behavior. However, since I'd begun reading and understanding, this behavior no longer made me upset. I learned to involve her in a favorite activity or to ask her to join me. She loved helping me. **Now I know that these activities made her feel appreciated.**

HOW DO YOU GET THEM TO EAT AND PLAY

THEN - 2008

I said "Oh, my gosh, She's having trouble chewing and swallowing. What should I do? Oh, I can prepare her food with a blender. I can give her baby food..." My mom didn't want anything to do with baby food or a food blender. So I learned how to cook soft food.

I knew not to rush my mom since I eat slowly myself. Oh yes, silently I said, "Are you kidding? You can't swallow chicken broth?" So I began giving her cold drinks with her meals. Oh yes, to finish this setting, I would give her a straw for her convenience.

What's wrong with this table setting?

NOW - 2010

Cold drinks are now easier for the patient to swallow.
Straws may cause additional swallowing problems.
Thin liquids such as coffee, tea or broth are hardest to swallow.
Caregivers may use a teaspoon of ice cream or sherbet to thicken liquids.
Planning and presenting soft, tasty, and healthy food makes sense to me.
Add Sprite or Ginger Ale to juices - especially Cranberry Juice. It's delicious!
Alzheimer patients do not like to be rushed. Remember Patience for the Patients.

Resources:
Caring for a Person with Alzheimer's Disease
The National Institute on Aging

THEN - 2008

Music, gardening, laundry, game shows, favorite television programs, housekeeping, and shopping were the extent of my suggested activities for the patient.

NOW - 2010

Card games, photography, jigsaw puzzles, car washing, and word games have been added to my list of activities patients, families and caregivers find rewarding.

In the **ALZHEIMER ACTIVITY GUIDE, Draw the Word** was particularly fascinating. This is a fun way to match words with pictures. For example, in this game, the patient could match the word *boy, cat, baby* with the picture, or the patient could draw the boy, the cat or the baby while the caregiver guessed what was being drawn. All of these activities are to be adjusted to the patient's level of ability. We all remember different versions of the game.

Resources:
In it Together
The Alzheimer's Activities Guide
Forest Pharmaceuticals, Inc.

14

THE CALM AFTER THE STORM

HOW CAN I GET THEM TO EAT AND PLAY?

I CAN ACCEPT THE THING I CAN'T CHANGE;
I CAN CHANGE THE THINGS I CAN CHANGE.

I CAN ASK FOR WISDOM TO UNDERSTAND WHAT I CAN'T CHANGE AND WHAT I CAN CHANGE.

I CAN FEEL SAD, SCARED, MAD, HAPPY.

I CAN SEE THAT GLASS AS HALF FULL INSTEAD OF HALF EMPTY.

I CAN FALL DOWN AND GET UP AGAIN- AND AGAIN- AND AGAIN AND...

I CAN HAVE COURAGE, LAUGHTER AND SERENITY.

I CAN HAVE FUN.

I CAN PLAN CALMING TREATS WITH ICE CREAM, JELL-O OR PUDDING.

A COOL TREAT THAT'S IN THE BAG
A FUN ACTIVITY

FOR EACH 2.5 CUP SERVING:
- Pour 1 cup whole milk in a small Ziploc plastic bag. Add 1 teaspoon of vanilla flavor and 1 tablespoon of sugar. Seal the bag.
- Place 12 ice cubes in a large Ziploc plastic bag. Sprinkle about 2 tablespoons of Salt on the cubes. Place the smaller bag inside the larger bag and seal the larger Bag.
- Everyone can take turns vigorously shaking the bag. Ice crystals should form in The milk mixture in about 10 minutes. When it begins to look like soft serve ice cream, scoop it out of the small bag. Add your favorite toppings and enjoy.

(A PERFECT TREAT AND ACTIVITY FOR PATIENTS AND CHILDREN)

HOW TO SURVIVE THE STORMS
1. Calm down and open your mind to the experience.
2. Accept and adopt a positive attitude.

QUESTION - WHAT IS A POSITIVE ATTITUDE?
ANSWER - We cannot change our past.

We cannot change the fact that people will act in a certain way. The only thing we can change is our attitude.
I frequently ask myself - Is this something I can change?
If the answer is "yes," I work diligently to change it.
If the answer is "no," I work diligently to accept it.

I GIVE TO THE WORLD THE BEST I HAVE AND THE BEST COMES BACK TO ME.

I FOLLOW THE GOLDEN RULE AND DO UNTO OTHERS AS I WOULD HAVE THEM DO UNTO ME.

I PURSUE THE SERENITY PRAYER DAILY:
I ask my Higher Power for the courage to change the things I can change.
I ask for the serenity to accept the things I cannot change.
I ask for the wisdom to know the difference.

QUESTION - SO WHAT IS THE HIGHER FORM OF LIVING YOU REFERRED TO IN THE PREFACE OF YOUR BOOK? HOW CAN WE JOIN?
ANSWER - I calm down and open my mind to the experience.
I accept and adopt a positive attitude.
I don't worry about the past because I can't change the past.
I accept the fact that people will act in a certain way.
I understand that the only thing I can change is my attitude.
I give to the world the best I have and the best is restored unto me.
I FOLLOW THE GOLDEN RULE AND I ADOPT THE SERENITY PRAYER

15

PICKING UP THE PIECES

RECONCILING YOUR DIFFERENCES

NO, PICKING UP the pieces is not about divorce or separation. In this chapter, I will pick up the pieces of several chapters, place the contents in one beautiful box, tie a ribbon on it and call it a gift.

THE DIVORCE

According to AARP, a controversial new theory gaining momentum in the scientific community, is that the brain is not destroyed by sticky plaque but by free floating clumps of protein. This AARP Bulletin arrived in my mailbox in September, 2010.

Coincidentally, I attended a conference on Alzheimer in early October, 2010. During the question and answer period, this discrepancy was very diplomatically revealed to the program providers. They either had not heard of this news or they did not acknowledge that it existed. Neither did they admit that this article may be worthy of further consideration

"Plaque is no longer where the action is."

Sam Gandy, M.D., at the Alzheimer's Disease Research Center at Mt. Sinai School of Medicine in New York, has been moving toward this theory for several years. If this theory is correct, then drugs that target plaque may not help people who have the disease. This research may comprise key information because approximately 5 million Americans have Alzheimer.

This is an exciting development!

William Thies, the Alzheimer's Association chief medical officer, cautions that Gandy's experiments need to be duplicated by other scientists in other labs before drug companies invest billions of dollars to create new medicines to target the clumps of protein in the brain.

In plain English, whether the brain cell is destroyed by plaque in one area of the brain or by clumps in the nearby area - who cares? Well, scientists care. Have scientists been going in the wrong direction for 20 years? Yes, we care. However, early-stage Alzheimer patients, family members and caregivers care most about the cure. Is it plaque or is it clumps? Let's target the right enemy.

WEDDING INVITATION RECONCILIATION

Scientists and Researchers:

You are invited to join hands and join research in the development of a whole new approach to finding a cure for Alzheimer. It is not about who is right and who is wrong. I know both sides of the family have worked separately to make the research a success. This offer expires at the end of 2013.

Please reconsider and accept this second invitation.

Sincerely yours,
Anne

"The best drugs are yet to come."

Rudolph Tanzi - (Director of Genetics and Aging Research Unit) compares the first Alzheimer drugs to a 10-year-old child shooting a soccer ball from mid-field: "Now we've got a division-one college team driving down the field."

Elizabeth Agnvall
AARP Contributing Editor

SOLVING THE PUZZLE AND FINDING THE CURE

Let's continue picking up the pieces. This is my unscientific solution to solving the puzzle and finding the solution. Yes, as I stated earlier, scientists must get on the same page. What's that buzz word? Yes - **collaborate** -

There are two clues in the Concentration Puzzle that must be turned over if you have the right information.

It is my unscientific but intellectual opinion that the symptoms have been verified for over

20 years, that the research has been proved and disproved for years. **Now is the time for all good men to come to the aid of their country.** I remembered this quote from over 20 years ago when self help booklets tried to teach me how to type. But I digress. **Now is the time for all good scientists to come to the aid of their country and find the cure for Alzheimer!**

Yes, thanks for entering my world. You want to know the second clue that is paramount to solving the puzzle - this Alzheimer puzzle?

Clue # two is caregivers.

Researchers, Scientists, Administrators, Authors, Aging networks, Alzheimer Support Groups, let's get together and involve the caregivers in your research and in your conferences. Involve them as expert witnesses.

This is more than comradeship!

This is that missing link - that missing clue that needs to be revisited

The caregiver is in there day and night - interacting with the Alzheimer patient through all phases of the disease. The caregiver is the one observing unique behaviors that have never been reported to researchers.

THE AMERICAN MEDICAL ASSOCIATION FAMILY GUIDE

states that the earliest signs of dementia may be so subtle that even the most perceptive physician fails to notice them. More often it is an observant relative or employer who first becomes aware of a certain lack of initiative, forgetfulness, and irritability on the part of the afflicted person.

Whatever the cause, a consistent approach to treatment will be necessary. Caregivers can provide observable behavioral changes in patients for the required consistent approach to treatments.

5.1 million Americans with Alzheimer's is unacceptable!

I believe that hundreds of caregivers representing thousands of Alzheimer patients can provide this link to the cure. We need local and state conferences, not only highlighting research and science, but also **highlighting the caregivers and what they can contribute to finding the cure.**

DIARY OF AN ALZHEIMER PATIENT — LESSONS I HAVE LEARNED

Most characteristic of dementia at the onset is the gradual loss of memory, especially for recent events although patients can recall what happened many years ago. As weeks and months pass, powers of reasoning and understanding dwindle. And there also may be a loss of interest in simple activities such as seeking news of relatives or friends.

This dementia often includes an emotional and physical instability. Mood swings between tears and laughter come at the slightest provocation. Odd, unpredictable quirks in behavior often become apparent as do uninhibited and anti-social actions. Table manners may deteriorate, personal cleanliness is sometimes neglected, and usual politeness abandoned. Some people may even become violent if impulsive behavior is questioned. I learned this lesson months after I began my care giving career. I wrongly characterized this behavior as due to old age. This means I believed the patient could improve his behavior

Apraxic disorders (in which there is an inability to coordinate muscles and movements), and aberrations of space perception may also be seen in severe cases due to Alzheimer disease. **In advanced stages of dementia, there is generalized stiffness of the muscles with slowness and awkwardness in all movements.** I observed this symptom with several patients; however, recently I applied my knowledge to the disease.

Toward the end, the affected person may have lost all ability to think, speak or move. This gradual collapse of the intellectual capabilities and emotions may linger on for ten years unless advance age or illness is present.

It is amazing how much I have learned since I began writing this book. You remember I described myself as a voracious reader.

Before my mom's diagnosis of Alzheimer in 2007, I would notice odd behavior:
- Burying all of the junk mail
- Covering all the mirrors when it thundered or rained
- Taping most of the light switches in the home
- Crying because she broke a glass or a plate
- Laughter at inappropriate times
- Being afraid of the thunder, the wind, and the rain.

In 2009 - two years after the diagnosis, I noticed - true to symptoms mentioned - that my mom lost interest in talking to one of her oldest friends even though she would communicate with the other three friends.

She did not become violent when her behavior was questioned, but she would become loud and say, "You all are so cruel to me." This happened each time she refused to take medications or go to the doctor when she'd fallen... Well, guess who bore the brunt of most of this abuse?

DEAR ANNIE,

All the letters are addressed to ANN with an 'E' - thus Dear Anne because the 'I' has been omitted from my name for over 20 years. Today, I am proud to insert the letter 'I'.

I deliberately saved the following letter to be used in this chapter...

I believe many of Americans need to pick up the pieces and live life more peacefully and more honestly. In a symbolic gesture, I am picking up the piece to my original name.

Here is the letter:

Dear Annie,

My mom has lived with me for two years in my home. Both my sister and I have been taking care of her. She has been diagnosed as a second-stage Alzheimer patient. She is presently living with my brother. I told him that either he takes her or she is going to the nursing home. For the past six months she has been fighting my sister and me. Two months ago, she decided to take up cursing. She cursed me every day for the last four weeks. She has called me all kinds of names. I don't think I can forgive her for this. **Sometimes, I really do hate my mom.**

DEAR CARRIE ANNE,

I understand your frustration and your attitude. Don't you want to feel better? Oh yes, I am going to tell you to read my book from cover to cover. However, first, I want you, your sister and your brother to seek out and join different support groups in the area. If they will not go, the only person you have complete control of is you.

Promise me that you will join one of these groups within the month. I am so sorry that you did not know about these support groups while your mom was staying with you and your sister. Read all the materials the group leader recommends, especially THE 36-HOUR DAY by Nancy L. Mace, M.A. and Peter Rabbins, M.D. This book is available in libraries and stores everywhere. Grand Central Publishing, a division of Hachette Book Group USA, Inc. is the publisher.

You may want to visit their website at www.HachetteBookGroupUSA.com. **Phone the Special Markets Department toll free at 1-800-222-6747. Fax: 1-800-477-5925.** Corporations and Organizations may purchase this book at quantity discounts. The 36-Hour Day has been revised and updated since 1984. I highly recommend this book.

The famous advice columnist, Ann Landers, in writing to a divorced couple says it so succinctly. "Hatred is like acid. It does more damage to the vessel in which it is stored than the object on which it is poured."

I know that you do not want your body, your mind, or your heart damaged.

Please write to me after you read the book and let me know how you are doing.

I care.

ANNIE

16

THIRTY-THREE LESSONS I HAVE LEARNED

1. BE THE FIRST TO SAY HELLO.

2. AN ARGUMENT CAN'T TAKE PLACE UNLESS TWO PEOPLE PARTICIPATE.

3. WHEN YOU DON'T KNOW FOR CERTAIN, GIVE THE PATIENT THE BENEFIT OF THE DOUBT.

4. TREAT THE PATIENT LIKE YOU WISH TO BE TREATED.

5. DON'T FRET THE SMALL STUFF.

6. LET SLEEPING DOGS LIE!

7. THE PATIENT'S GREATEST EMOTIONAL NEED IS TO BE APPRECIATED AND FEEL VALUED.

8. GIVE TO THE WORLD THE BEST YOU HAVE AND THE BEST WILL COME BACK TO YOU.

9. IF YOU GIVE AND EXPECT SOMETHING IN RETURN, IT IS NOT A GIFT; IT IS A TRADE.

10. PATIENTS NEED OUR PATIENCE.

AUTOBIOGRAPHY IN FIVE SHORT CHAPTERS

1
I WALK DOWN THE STREET.
THERE IS A DEEP HOLE IN THE SIDEWALK.
I FALL IN
I AM LOST. I AM HELPLESS
IT ISN'T MY FAULT.
IT TAKES FOREVER TO FIND MY WAY OUT.

2
I WALK DOWN THE SAME STREET.
THERE IS A DEEP HOLE IN THE SIDEWALK.
I PRETEND I DON'T SEE IT.
I FALL IN AGAIN.
I CAN'T BELIEVE I AM IN THE SAME PLACE
BUT IT ISN'T MY FAULT.
IT STILL TAKES A LONG TIME TO GET OUT.

3
I WALK DOWN THE SAME STREET.
THERE IS A DEEP HOLE IN THE SIDEWALK.
I SEE IT IS THERE
I STILL FALL IN...IT'S A HABIT.
MY EYES ARE OPEN.
I KNOW WHERE I AM.
IT IS MY FAULT.
I GET OUT IMMEDIATELY.

4
I WALK DOWN THE SAME STREET.
THERE IS A DEEP HOLE IN THE SIDEWALK.
I WALK AROUND IT.

5
I WALK DOWN ANOTHER STREET.

LETTING GO

I HAVE LEARNED TO LET GO.

TO LET GO IS NOT TO CUT MYSELF OFF; IT'S KNOWING I CAN'T CONTROL OTHER PEOPLE.

TO LET GO IS NOT TRYING TO CHANGE OTHERS. WE CAN ONLY CHANGE US.

TO LET GO IS NOT TO DENY, BUT TO ACCEPT.

TO LET GO IS NOT TO SCOLD, ARGUE, OR CORRECT OUR PATIENTS, BUT TO SEARCH FOR WAYS TO IMPROVE US.

TO LET GO IS NOT TO FIX, BUT TO BE SUPPORTIVE.

TO LET GO IS NOT TO ADJUST EVERYTHING TO OUR DESIRES, BUT TO CHERISH THE MOMENT.

TO LET GO IS NOT TO REGRET THE PAST, BUT TO IMPROVE IN THE FUTURE.

TO LET GO IS TO FEAR LESS AND TO LOVE MORE.

TO LET GO IS NOT TO JUDGE BUT TO BECOME HUMAN AGAIN.

I HAVE LEARNED
That if someone says something unkind about me,
I must live so that no one believes it.

I HAVE LEARNED
That silent company is often more healing than words of advice.
That life sometimes gives you a second chance.

I HAVE LEARNED
That if you pursue happiness, it will elude you.
But if you focus on your family, the needs of others,
And doing the best you can,
Happiness will find you.

I HAVE LEARNED
That wherever I go - the world's worst drivers have followed me there!

I HAVE LEARNED
That whenever I decide something with kindness,
I usually make the right decision.

I HAVE LEARNED
That there are people who love you dearly
But just don't know how to show it.

I HAVE LEARNED
That each day we should reach out and touch someone.
People love that human touch - holding hands - a warm hug,
Or just a friendly pat on the back.

I HAVE LEARNED
That sooner or later, all the people
Of the world will have to discover
A way to live together in peace...
If this is to be achieved, man

Must evolve for all human conflict
A method which rejects revenge,
Aggression, and retaliation.

**The foundation
Of such a method is love.
Dr. Martin Luther King Jr.**

I HAVE LEARNED
That I still have a lot to learn...

APPENDIX

DICTIONARY DIRECTORY

ABC

ALZHEIMER

She has Alzheimer disease

She has a medical condition that affects the brain and causes significant memory loss, poor judgment, confusion, anxiety, frequent or sudden changes in mood or behavior and loss of interest in activities previously enjoyed.

CLINICAL TRIAL

Has he participated in a clinical trial?

A clinical trial is a research study to find out if new medications or treatments are safe and effective.

ADEAR

Please call the ADEAR Center.

ADEAR Centers publish books about Alzheimer's Disease (ADEA) - 1-800-438-4380

DEF

Delusions

She has delusions.

She has false beliefs that she believes are real.

DEMENTIA
Oh, he is suffering from dementia
Dementia describes the Alzheimer group of symptoms listed earlier.

DNR
Has she signed a DNR form?
A document that tells health care staff how the person wants end-of-life care managed.

GH

HALLUCINATIONS
Does he suffer from hallucinations?
Does he see, hear, smell, taste or feel something that is not there?

I

INCONTINENT
Is she incontinent?
Does she have trouble controlling her bowels or bladder?

JKL

LIVING WILL
He has a living will in his safe deposit box at the bank.
A legal document that states a person's wishes for end-of-life care.

MNO

MEDICAID
Does she qualify for Medicaid or Medicare?
A Federal and State Government health care program for low-income families.

MEDICARE
A Federal Government health insurance plan that pays some costs for people 65 and older.

PQR

PACE

Did you enroll him in PACE?

PACE combines Medicaid and Medicare benefits to help older people stay at home.

ST

TIA: TRANSIENT ISCHEMIC ATTACK

A temporary impairment of brain function due to an insufficient supply of blood to part of the brain. She may have slurred speech, dizziness or nausea. She may be weak or paralyzed. The symptoms last only a few minutes or a few hours, then the patient recovers.

UVW

WANDER OR WANDERING

Has he started wandering?

Is there a constant pacing

To go from place to place in an agitated or aimless way; ramble or roam

APPENDIX II

A CAREGIVER'S BILL OF RIGHTS

I have the right:
- To take care of me, myself and I.
- To ask assistance from others even when the patient may object. See #1 above.
- To refrain from placing my entire life on hold. See #1 above.
- To get angry, express anger, be depressed and feel guilty occasionally.
- To receive acceptance and affection for my service.
- To prepare for my future when my patient will not need my assistance full-time.
- To expect and demand that we find new resources for the caregivers.

Modified by Today's Caregiver magazine

CAREGIVER'S BILL OF RIGHTS
- Caregivers have the right to receive sufficient training in care giving skills and understandable information about the condition of the patient.
- Caregivers have the right to receive appreciation and emotional support from male and female family members.
- Caregivers have the right to provide for care at home or in a care facility.
- Caregivers have the right to expect professionals to be knowledgeable about options related to the patient and the caregivers.
- Caregivers have the right to supportive employers when dealing with the unexpected or serious care needs of the patient.

APPENDIX III

POEMS

IT COULDN'T BE DONE

By Edgar A. Guest

There are thousands to tell you it cannot be done,
There are thousands to prophesy failure;
There are thousands to point out to you, one by one,
The danger that waits to assail you.
But just buckle in with a bit of a grin,
Just take off your coat and go to it,
Just start to sing as you tackle the thing
That "cannot be done," and you'll do it.

ODE TO THE CURE

By A. Gaskins Laws

There are dozens to whisper it cannot be done.
There are dozens to predict failure;
There are dozens to point out to you, one by one,
The cure that waits to fail you.
So just wander in with a bit of a grin,
Just take off your shoes and research it,
Just begin to write as you choose to ignite
That "cannot be done" and you'll do it.

ATTITUDE

The longer I live, the more I understand the effect of my attitude on my life. Attitude to me is more important than what other people think, than what other people say, than what other people do. Attitude is more important than the past. I cannot change my past, I cannot change the fact that people will act in a certain way. The only thing I can change is my attitude. I am convinced that my life is about 10% what happens to me and about 90% what mind set I adapt and what attitude I adopt.

ATTITUDE

I promise myself...

To think only of the best, to work only for the best, and to expect only the best will come back to me. I promise to forget the mistakes of the past and to expect from myself greater achievements in the future. I promise that I will spend so much time improving myself that I will not have time to criticize and ridicule others. I promise myself that I will always look at that glass as half full and make this optimism come true in my life. I promise to be too busy for worry, too noble for anger, too strong for fear, and too happy to permit the presence of trouble...because my attitude is my life.

EDUCATION AND RESOURCES

MANY NATIONAL ORGANIZATIONS have local or state chapters. Ask for their state listing or check your telephone directory for a local listing.

Alzheimer's Disease Education and Referral Center (ADEAR)
P.O. Box 8250
Silver Springs, Md. 20907-8250
Toll-free - 1-800-438-4350
www.nia.nih.gov/Alzheimers

Alzheimer's National Association - www.alz.org
Alzheimer's National Toll-free 24-hour Help Line - 1-800-272-3900

Alzheimer's Store - www.alzstore.com
Alzheimer's Store - 1-800-752-3238

Dementia USA:
www.dementiausa.com

Learning to Speak Alzheimer's: by Joanne Koenig Coste
www.learningtospeakAlzheimer.com

Medic Alert + Safe Return
2323 Colorado Avenue Turlock, CA 95382

1-888-572-8566
www.medicalert.org/safereturn

National Hospice Organization
1901 N. Moore St., Suite 901
Arlington, Va. 22209
Toll-free - 1-800-65 8-8898
http://www.nho.org

National Institute of Health; National Institute of Neurological Disorders and Stroke; Brain Basics; http:inds.nih.gov/disorders/brain-basics-know-your-brain.htm
The 36 Hour Day by Nancy Mace, M.A. and Peter Rabins, MD.
Published by the John Hopkins University Press, 1981.

A COOL TREAT
(THAT'S IN THE BAG)

FOR EACH 2 ½ CUP SERVING:
- Pour 1-cup whole milk in a small Ziploc plastic bag. Add 1 teaspoon of vanilla flavor and 1 tablespoon of sugar. Seal the bag.
- Place 12 ice cubes in a large Ziploc plastic bag. Sprinkle about 2 tablespoons of Salt on the cubes. Place the smaller bag inside the larger bag and seal the larger Bag.
- Everyone can take turns vigorously shaking the bag. Ice crystals should form in the milk mixture in about 10 minutes. When it begins to look like soft serve ice cream, scoop it out of the small bag. Add your favorite toppings and enjoy.